MW00478101

ISBN-10: 1478200561
ISBN-13: 978-1478200567

Introduction to Image Medicine.
Outlined in Russian by Tamara Martynova.
Translated from Russian
M.: "Sophia," 2011.—48 p. Series "Enter your inner world"

Translator: Margarita A. Bronshteyn, skyblue41325@gmail.com

INTRODUCTION TO IMAGE MEDICINE

MINGTANG XU

Image medicine belongs to an ancient Chinese branch of medicine that attempts to uncover the mysteries of the human body with all its functions and systems, the meaning of life as a whole, and the qualities of an image. It dives into the effects of images on a human as an integrated system composed of a physical body, an energy system, and informational system.

In this book, the reader is briefly introduced to the philosophical concepts behind the origin of images of a human and the universe as well as the practical application of these images in the realm of energetic anatomy and physiology. Inside, you will find descriptions of the approaches needed to acquire the images necessary for diagnosis, treatment, and illness prevention. Suggested techniques of self healing as well as some Big Methods and mantras for the correction and restoration of numerous bodily functions are included in the text.

This book is intended for a wide range of readers; including medical field employees and Qigong practitioners.

Contents

FOREWORD

Image medicine (IM) belongs to an ancient Chinese branch of medicine and utilizes its approaches to correction and regulation of a person's health as holistic and integrated system.

This approach is one which explores the components of the human, the meaning of life, and the qualities of an image. This form of medicine is based on and utilizes the ability of the mind to operate images, or pictures.

Here we analyze the philosophical concepts concerning the origin of the world on the basis of images of the universe and of a human, as well as the questions concerning the acquisition, formulation, and influence of images on a person, including on his physical body, energy system, and informational system.

Today, IM can be applied to the scientific field. Research is being conducted on how such images can be used in the realms of diagnosis, treatment, and illness prevention. Furthermore, several important Big Methods and mantras have been found to help correct and regulate numerous bodily functions of a human as a life form.

Like in any form of medicine, anatomy and physiology are also researched. However, unlike the normal form of anatomy and physiology in which the physical structure and functions of the body are discussed, here we discuss the energy and informational systems of the human body. Therefore, in IM there exist several stages or parts. The first part is energetic medicine (energetic anatomy and physiology), the second part is information medicine (information anatomy and physiology), the third is substances, and the fourth is all of the aforementioned combined. As of today, only the first two are open: energetic medicine and information medicine.

It is important to note that the current division is not set in stone and, in practice, all the parts are applied in certain groupings and combinations.

For example, in the energetic part of IM one studies the locations, interactions, and functions of energetic canals, biologically active points, Dan Tian areas, and other energetic zones and structures of our body, as well as the functions and effects of fog energy, light energy, and transcendental energy.

In the subsequent books a detailed analysis of the methods of diagnosis and treatment as well as the theoretical backbone of each will be explored.

This form of medicine is based on and utilizes the ability of the mind to operate images or pictures.

SYNOPSIS OF THE ORIGIN OF IMAGE MEDICINE

The term "Image Medicine" stems from the translation of the Chinese phrase 意象医学 (read as "Yi Xiang Yi Xue"), in which:

意 "Yi" means mind, consciousness, and thoughts, (This hieroglyph is also used to describe any actions done by the mind.)

象 "Xiang" translates as pictures or images,

医 "Yi" means medicine,

学 "Xue" is interpreted as science.

How can one further understand the meaning of this phrase in the Chinese language? It means that one needs to think using his mind, thoughts, consciousness, and awareness. When we think about something, the action includes a conscious acknowledgement of our current, as well as future, actions. Meanwhile, there is a constant array of images that appear in our minds.

Image Medicine, combined with Traditional Chinese Medicine (TCM), can be considered a completed composition of ancient Chinese medicine. Due to certain historical events, some aspects of this medical knowledge, such as the actual use of images, have been lost in time, leaving only the names of some methods without any explanation or practical application.

Now, for example, in TCM pulse-diagnosis is called "mai xiang", which is literary translated into "the image of a pulse or a blood vessel". Currently, students in universities study how to sense a pulse, rather than see an image of it, even though the name of the practice has remained the same.

The part of Chinese Medicine called "Zan Xiang", the study of the manifestation of images, provides a detail-less description of work with images. However, a large portion of information from this part has been lost.

The origin of IM is rooted in the history of ancient China. Its founder is considered the Chinese doctor Bian Que, now honored as a saint in modern China. A lot of myths are associated with this revered doctor, one is as follows.

Once, Bian Que found himself in the capital of an empire whose prince was seriously ill. Walking by the imperial court, Chueh turned to the guards and asked them to pass on to the emperor that he could to treat the prince. The guards demanded proof that the doctor was not lying and could in fact cure their ill prince. Bian Que responded by saying that he needed to neither listen to the prince's pulse nor see the patient at all—Chueh could describe his symptoms to the guards right then and there. The doctor explained that the prince was suffering from heat in his leg and a twitching ear. The guards immediately informed the court of the unknown doctor and the emperor confirmed that those were the symptoms his son was suffering from. In this way, Bian Que was permitted into the palace and allowed to treat the prince.

Following the recovery of the prince, Bian Que was asked to stay by the palace where he continued to lead many investigations and to demonstrate diagnostic and treatment miracles. He had a reputation of an unusual doctor and other court doctors tremendously envied him. And what was the secret behind his successful treatments? Precisely that he was able to operate images.

One day, the emperor himself fell ill. None of the court doctors were able to cure him and were forced to turn to Bian Que for help. Once again, Chueh demonstrated healing miracles.

Sadly, shortly after healing the emperor, Bian Que was brutally murdered. In his honor and to demonstrate his gratitude for being cured, the emperor began compiling a book about Chinese medicine. Despite the fact that the book was written by the emperor, it generally presented all the medical knowledge the court doctors possessed. However, most of the knowledge and methods of Bian Que was not included in the book. It is now preserved solely through oral tradition and is mostly spoken of among village healers who continue to apply images to their healing.

The basis of Traditional Chinese Medicine stems from the emperors and several ancient dissertations. However, many terms mentioned in the dissertations of the Yellow Emperor Huang Dee lack explanations and thus their meanings are lost. Images, and their use in diagnostics, are often mentioned but the lack of ways to utilize these images makes their application impossible. Modern Chinese medical field employees are still hopeful that some of Bian Que's knowledge will one day be restored. Currently there exist two branches of Chinese medicine: that of the Yellow Emperor and that of Bian Que. The union of these two branches would mean the restoration of the complete form of Chinese Medicine.

Part One

BASICS OF IMAGE MEDICINE: THEORY AND PHILOSOPHY

Chapter One:
THE CONCEPT OF AN IMAGE

WHAT IS AN IMAGE?

An image is a picture that occurs within us, in our heads, as though on an internal screen. One can say that an image is a reflection of the universe and all the things within it. The material world around us can be represented as an image and all that can be seen or felt calls forth a particular image.

We can separate *external* and *internal images*.

Some people possess very strong and clear images while others have weaker ones. However, the later have other more developed senses such as improved hearing capabilities.

If the subject is viewed as a whole, then images (or pictures) or sounds are all the same—simply wave radiation or fluctuation. Only, images have a wider meaning whereas sounds evoke pictures of a more narrow meaning. A sound is a function of our hearing alone, but images are a function of our mind, our soul, and our sight. After some practice one can learn to transform sounds into images. This is relatively easy to do and with further practice one can also learn to see images of a companion's thoughts.

As a result we can see images. This ability explains why when you look at something you receive an image of that which you see. Also, it means that if you hear my voice then you can create an image of me in your mind.

And so we have determined that by utilizing our normal sensory organs we can receive images. This means that everything in the outer world can be reflected as an image in our brain and thus is called an external image.

A viewer can receive such an image through the help of sight. In this case, a picture that reflects the outside world forms in a person's mind. This picture is not a true depiction of the object but rather an image of it. Thus, if one looks at himself in the mirror, the reflection is not the true portrayal of the person but rather, once again, an image of him.

In the process of thinking an array of images constantly appear in a person's mind. The material world around us can be converted into images and the sensations from various organs provide different images (Picture 1).

Hearing. Sounds that a person registers through the use of hearing capabilities can be translated into images. Hearing a familiar voice can produce an image of the person to whom the voice belongs in the listener's mind. The sound of heavy wind

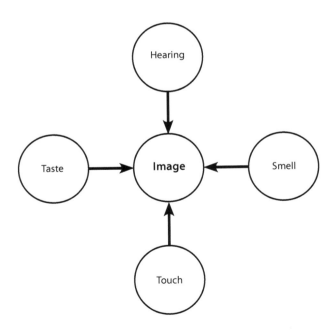

Picture 1: The Formation of Images through Different Sensory Organs

and rain can be transformed into an image of trees shaking under the strong wind gusts.

Touch. Touching produces particular sensations: warm, cold, rough, smooth, etc. through feeling a particular object a person can produce an image of the object in his mind. A stranger's touch can also call forth a particular image. The degree of the correctness and reality of the image often depends on the imagination of a person.

Smell. Smelling organs also help produce certain images. A person can sense a smell as he passes by a bakery and automatically the image of fresh loaves of bread appears in his mind.

Taste. Taste receptors help determine what us being consumed and thus cause the mind to form an image of the meal.

And so, *with the help of any of the organs, a person receives images. Thus, all external things are reflected in the observer's brain and become transformed into external images by the observer.* However, it is important to note that *an image and reality are two different concepts.*

A person has the ability to receive images but may experience difficulty understanding reality.

Let's look at an example. Looking at me, an observer sees black hair, that is, he receives an image of black hair. However, how can he be sure that my hair is black? In other words, how realistic is this image? We know that under the sun's rays the hair gives the impression of being black, but in darkness hair cannot be seen at all and under a red light the hair would acquire a different shade. Thus it can be said that the image received in the presents of sunlight happens to be *relative*, not real and not *absolute*. An image is rooted in its surroundings, that is, in a standard setting the observer receives a particular image. Henceforth, it can be said that all knowledge is in fact relative and not absolute. Due to this everything that a person knows about the world around him is but an image rather than reality or truth.

Another example is as follows. Several people are looking at a flower from different sides and are receiving a particular image of the flower depending on which side they are observing from. The flower could be drawn or photographed but in either case the picture would not be of a flower since every vantage point looks upon only a portion of the flower rather than at the flower from the inside out. The receiving of the image relies on the actual flower, the eyes of the onlooker, and the surroundings. Each representation of the picture can be different but each picture portrays this flower. This is the image.

An *internal image* is an image that forms in the mind of a person as a result of thinking, imagining, dreaming, visualizing, etc. without any disturbances to sensory organs. *An example:* You are sitting with your eyes closed smiling because you have a date with a pretty girl (or with a young man). Thoughts about this date are causing certain images to appear in your mind. This means that you can produce an image in your mind without being influenced by sensations from the external world. This also means that understanding of the external occurs through internal perception.

The result of the aforementioned is that absolutely every part of our body, absolutely every part of the external world can be reflected internally in the form of an image. *The external world produces internal images that we can then send into the external surroundings.* Thus, to understand anything outside the body, a human has to utilize his sensory organs.

Here, when we discuss understanding, we assume that the "creation of an image within us" is the receiving of definite information. An image does not reveal itself as a true external object in the full meaning of the word. This is similar to looking at yourself in the mirror and receiving only a reflection, your image, rather than a true portrayal yourself. Thus, through interactions with the outside world, we receive internal images as a result of the work of our sensory organs. With this, every part of our physical body allows for the receiving and understanding of images and every internal organ, every inner part of the body, has its own image within our mind.

Analyze the opposing situation: how are internal images going to affect on the physical body, the functions of the organs, and the behavior of a person?

Every person dreams dreams but what is a dream? Basically, it is the work of our brain, our mind, which produces a many pictures as we sleep. Our body can lie in a bed but meanwhile our consciousness is running through image of us being in an unlimited amount of places and situations. If you fall in your dream, your body shudders and you awake with the recollection of the dream. While you were asleep, no one was sending you images, you were asleep and did not see the surrounding environment. However, the brain still creates images within us.

An example. You are dreaming of something very sad and are, as a result, crying. You are crying in your dream but wake up to find that you had actually physically cried as well and your face was now wet from tears.

These examples demonstrate that internally produced images have a direct and profound effect on both our physical body as well as on our behavior. Furthermore, *an image, created in the mind of an onlooker without any distractions from the sensory organs, we will refer to as mental images.*

WHAT IS IMAGE MEDICINE?

Image Medicine is a system that allows one to understand the components of a human and the meaning of life as a whole. In reality, every living form around us is nothing more or less than an image. We create images, we receive images, and these images impact our lives.

IM is one branch of science that investigates the effects of particular images on parts or organs of the body as well as explores the application of images as a method to correct and regulate functions of the entire physical body, including its energetic and informational systems.

It is exceptionally difficult to understand this science as a whole. It is only possible to process this science one step at a time, slowly immersing yourself in it and perfecting your mastery of it. For example, an image affects our physical body through the application of energy. We know that energy has a profound effect on our physical bodies but how exactly does this effect occur?

First off, it is linked to the images that already exist within us. For example, a person looks at another and receives an image that the later will be involved in a car accident. Or you can receive an image that one of your friends will pay you a visit and this in fact happens. At this point you begin to understand that *you first receive an image and then something occurs in reference to this image.* Thus, when you observe a bud blossoming, you may receive an image of a future leaf on the steam. At this time the leaf is still very small but the image will be of a fully-formed, large leaf. Similarly, you can receive an image of a patient becoming ill and, if you change the image, you can cause the disease to disappear. We can say that an image refers to an internal reflection and *real life is fully dependent on these images*. We attempt to comprehend the images and in turn use them to regulate our lives. By changing the images we can change our lives.

If an image is originally wrong it means that at some age in the person's life he will fall ill. We can learn to check images in order to determine the likelihood of future illness. Similarly, we can check the images of a patient for signs of illness.

As a whole, images are primary aspects of one's life and are linked to the person, his soul, his spirit, and his energy. First images appear and only after are information, energy, and physical wellbeing processed. If there is no person there can be no images and before human existence there were no images since images are but a reflection of the outside world within one's mind. This means that if we can regulate and change images then we can control our spirit, our energy, and our body.

In Chinese culture there is music produced on special instruments based on the theory of Wu-Xing (five elements). When we listen to music, we receive an image that then affects our body.

There is a therapy that applies the use of pictures in order to treat a patient. The patient is asked to look at pictures and, following the procedure, his illness simply disappears. Many images are used during this treatment. We show the patient particular imaged and, in turn, the images work within the patient's body. In IM we attempt to understand the essence of life and, when we look deeper, we discover that particular images play a vital role in it from the start. We create images, we receive images, and these images impact our lives.

It is important to understand that images are three-dimensional pictures. Unlike physical eyes that can only observe in one direction, images can be observed from different direction, and not only can their surfaces be viewed but also they can be viewed from the inside as well. This kind of sight is called "The Eye of the Mind", or "The Eye of the Heart". For this, in order to see an image, one needs a calm body and a silent mind.

Chapter Two:
DEVELOPMENT OF LIFE
AND MODELS OF A HUMAN

THE ORIGIN OF LIFE

Medicine, above all, applies to life and thus it is vital to understand what life is. An image is an effective investigative tool that can show what life is and how it develops. Ancient Chinese texts describe a concept on the development of life through images received by a person's mind while in a state of deep meditation (Picture 2).

The primordial image is impossible to describe and it simply named Tao. Furthermore, Tao created Emptiness, which, in this context, does not mean the complete absence of anything, but rather the simultaneous existence and nonexistence of everything. Emptiness, in turn, created two forms of energy: Yin and Yang (one active, the other passive). Yin-Yang then created the

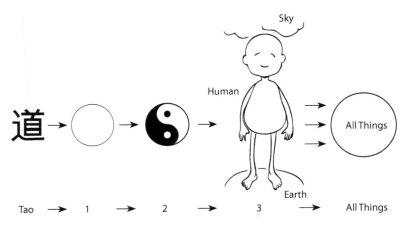

Picture 2: The Evolution of the Universe and Origin of Life According IM

10

Sky, the Earth, and the Human. Tao, Emptiness, and Yin-Yang are all verbal descriptions of images that are processed by the mind and not by the regular sight of the observer. These images mean that on the outside, a human is linked to the Sky and the Earth while on the inside, a human is similar to the Universe and has the same three components: physical, energetic, and information (more about these components will come in future sections).

From this theory on the development of the world, one can see that images describe and determine the principles or rules of the evolution of life. While in the state of Emptiness, the Universe possesses an image, Yin-Yang has an image, and the current situation as a whole has an image. For all the manifested and non-manifested there is an image.

A MODEL OF THE UNIVERSE

The basic theory of IM explains what life is, what a human is, and what the universe is. IM also provides a model of the universe which states that the universe was formed with the help of matter, energy, and information. As in the life of an individual, the universe, too, was formed with the help of images.

The universe's energy can be divided into three subcategories based on the functions of the energy. The first is referred to as fog energy because it looks like fog. When we say "looks like" it means that it produces an image of fog within us. The second subcategory is the energy of light. This type of energy produces an image (or picture) of multicolored light. Lastly, the third type of energy is called transcendental energy. It does not produce any concrete image but rather it produces an image of Emptiness. (Picture 3)

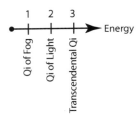

Picture 3: Graphical Depiction
of Energy Aspect

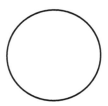

Picture 4: The Image
of Emptiness

The physical world can also be divided into three parts or three levels: one-dimensional, two-dimensional, and three-dimensional. We can observe these levels or parts with the help of images. A one-dimensional space looks like a point or a line (Picture 4). A two-dimensional space calls forth an image of a plane (Picture 5). Lastly, we live in a three-dimensional space (Picture 6). Likewise, we understand that the world in composed of matter and that the substances in our world also produce certain images.

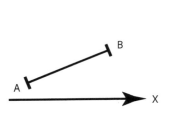

Picture 5: Graphical Image
of One-dimensional World

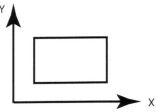

Picture 6: Graphical Image
of Two-dimensional World

The information aspect of the universe can also be divided into three parts: Yin-information, Yuan-information, and Yang-information (Picture 7).

By examining this model, it becomes evident that ***everything can be reflected as a picture composed of three axes: matter (or space), energy, and information*** (Picture 8). Since every

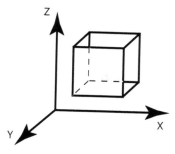

Picture 7: Graphical Image
of Tree-dimensional World

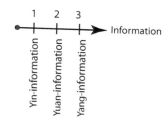

Picture 8: Graphical Depiction
of Informational Aspect

axis, or part, is composed of three subcategories (described above), then in total we have $3*3*3 = 27$ variations which are characteristic of 27 different images or levels of worlds (Picture 9).

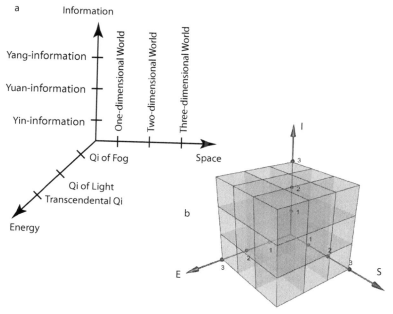

Picture 9: The Model of the Universe (a) Three Components, or Aspects, (b) Twenty Seven Images, or Levels of the Worlds

13

The world below us consists of two space dimensions but possesses a spirit developed to the level of Yang-shen and an energy developed to the transcendental level. From the bottom, it is the eighteenth (3*3*2) world. Therefore, our world is the nineteenth in succession. This means that below us there exist eighteen worlds and above us there are eight worlds.

In Taoism it is confirmed that there exist eight levels of heaven and eighteen levels of hell. If we are able to leap even one world higher, we will acquire longevity and will be rid of suffering and sickness.

A MODEL OF A HUMAN

In the traditional Chinese philosophy and medicine, as well as in the theories of Qigong, it is considered that a human is a small universe. This means that we are like the big universe. As in, the amount of separate worlds in the universe corresponds with the amount of separate life functions within us.

The same three parts apply to the human existence as those that apply to the universe: the physical body, energy, and soul. The physical body, our physical composition, can be further divided into three parts. We can say that certain materials and functions in our body present images of life in the form of points and lines. These materials, this matter, we refer to as one-dimensional substances. Others provide images of planes and are named two-dimensional substances. And still others call forth three-dimensional images and are thus called three-dimensional substances.

The energy within us and everywhere else in the universe is exactly the same. Our energy divides into three types as well, in the same way as the energy of the universe is portioned.

Our soul can also be divided into three levels. The first level is simply the soul (in Chinese this is called Yin-shen). The

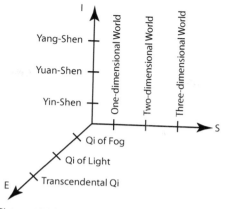

Picture 10: The Model of the Human

second level is Yuan-shen while the third level is Yang-shen (Picture 10).

If our physical body is examined as a holistic system and divided into parts, then we can identify 27 subsystems. For better understanding, this means that the human body is composed of nine functioning systems. Energy and spirit can likewise be divided into nine subsystems each. Therefore, this image must, above all, provide us with a model of the universe. Furthermore, it also provides us with an understanding of the relationship between the human and the universe.

A MODEL OF ILLNESSES

As a human we are composed of a physical body, energy, and spirit. What disruptions occur within us in the process of becoming ill?

During illness, there may be disruptions to the work of the physical body such as in the event of a broken bone, a knife wound, and so on. However, an illness can be brought on by problems with energy, for example as a result of excessive cold within the body. Pains in the body can occur in cases of blocked energetic channels; a low level of energy can cause a person to experience exhaustion even after resting; an excess of bad energy often brings about aggressiveness, constant quarreling with those around you, and a desire for a fight someone.

Problems can also arise with one's consciousness, mind, or spirit. When you hear bad news you may experience depression, or if there is something confusing occurring in your family you may feel frightened. Occasionally, a person experiences negative emotions that are then reinforced by stress for no apparent reason.

And so, illness can be physical, energetic, emotional, or spiritual. Often, an illness is composed of not one of these categories but combinations of two, sometimes even three, of them (Picture 11). For example, there can be problems with both physical and energetic aspects as well as illness of spiritual and energetic aspects and illness with physical and spiritual charac-

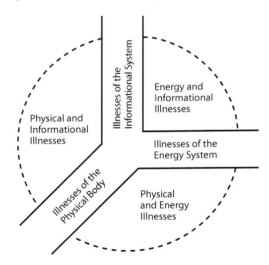

Picture 11: Different Categories of Illnesses

teristics. One of the manifestations of the last combination is constant fear. This phenomenon belongs to spiritual problems but, despite all your efforts, the fear does not go away. Why? This phenomenon occurs because on the physical level there are problems with the kidneys such as a disruption in their work or a withering away of part of a kidney. Everything is interconnected—the problem with the kidneys on a physical level and the fear on a spiritual level. Therefore, this requires solving the combined problem of both the spirit and physical body. Occasionally, an illness is the result of problems of all three parts, an illness of the physical body leads to the manifestation of problems with one's energy and spirit as well. For example, a stroke begins from problems on the energetic and physical planes but ultimately affects the spiritual plane as well by causing anger and aggression. Similarly, phenomena can be observed in the case of cancer as well.

Therefore, we must understand that disruptions in any constituent of our organism, whether physical, energetic, or information, undeniably affects the other components of our body (Picture 12).

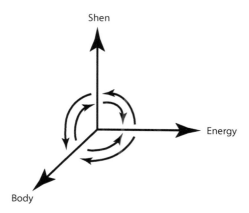

Picture 12: Interaction of Three Aspects of a Human

Therefore the following types of illnesses may occur:

- Illnesses of the physical body;
- Illnesses of the energy system;
- Illnesses of the informational system;
- Illnesses of an energy-informational character;
- Illnesses of a physical and energy plan;
- Physical and informational illnesses;
- Physical and energy-informational illnesses.

MODELS OF TREATMENT

IM presents itself as panoramic medicine. It explores and treats illness in terms of what constitutes life as whole. Since the treatments in IM use the combined effects of physical, energetic, and spiritual methods, we can say that it is a holistic and integrated system. Every doctor who implements the use of methods from IM must be able to operate all three components of the system equally well. Since the doctors are not divided into subcategories, following a diagnosis, a patient must be treated by one doctor. Therefore, for work as an image therapist it is imperative to master the treatment as a whole.

Treatment through IM is a completely natural form of treatment. It is a method through which one human being treats another. Usually we act as follows: we use our personal energy or our own mind to treat another. Of course, in certain situations it is imperative to also use special feeding, herbs, and other methods such as surgery. For example, a very famous ancient doctor Huat also implemented surgical practices alongside feeding, herbs, and methods of practice.

Treatment in IM is based on the concepts of the types of illnesses. Therefore, if we have seven separate groups of illnesses, then there should also be seven methods or groups of treating the illnesses:

- Physical Method
- Energy Method
- Spiritual Method
- Physical and Energy Method
- Physical and Spiritual Method
- Physical, Energy, and Spiritual Method

We will look at only one example and further analysis of other examples will come in subsequent books. *An Example:* Can we apply physical and energetic forms of healing to spiritual illnesses? Let us analyze an emotion such as fear. If someone is constantly experiencing fear then he is spiritually ill. How can physical methods of treatment be used to help cure this illness?

Fear, as a rule, is a symptom of certain kidney problems. We can use herbs for the strengthening of kidney functions as a method of treatment. Likewise, we can supply the patient with additional energy for the kidneys—an energetical treatment of a spiritual illness.

There exists one standard of health and countless amounts of deviations from this standard that present themselves as illnesses. Moreover, every year there are new illnesses, the research of which is complicated by the ever-growing amount of them. Despite the numerous investigations, the cause of many illnesses is still unknown and, henceforth, there is no proper treatment for them. In IM, image diagnostics are utilized, making it very easy to determine the condition of one's health.

PRINCIPLES OF DIAGNOSIS

Diagnosis with the help of images allows for an accurate evaluation of a person's health. If a person is healthy, the image will not change since a changing image is a symptom of illness. *For Example:* Looking at a tree, one can instantly decipher between old and new foliage or between a healthy and sick tree. A similar observation occurs upon the diagnosis of a human. If one knows how health presents itself, then it is not necessary to learn of all the illnesses. For example, even if a person has no knowledge about leaf illnesses, by looking at a leaf, he will still be able to determine whether or not it is healthy.

Image diagnosis allows one to understand the difference between health and illness. The value of an image is crucial in this case. An image of health is reminiscent of a clean and clear mirror, whereas the image of illness is a muddy, foggy, and dirty depiction of the injured area. This is similar to two cups of water, one clear and the other muddy.

As a whole, the diagnostic methods of IM allows one to discover an image of the illness while the treatment methods of IM is the transformation of incorrect images to correct ones— the transformation of an ill individual to a healthy one.

For better understanding and application, the theory and practice of IM is divided into several parts but only the first two, Energy medicine and Informational medicine, are available to study since the later parts are composed of secret knowledge possessed only by the masters.

In IM a certain form of diagnosis is implemented. Several methods can be utilized simultaneously but, at the end of the day, an illness must be identified through energetic, physical, and spiritual means. This means that we must have a method of identification of problems in, for example, a person's energy system. This is why the first form of diagnosis we implement is energetic diagnosis, which allows us to identify problems with a patient's energy system.

In the presents of a spiritual problem we must understand the feelings and sensations experienced by the patient. Emotional or spiritual problems in this sense mean that a person may feel frightened, depressed, alarmed, unsure, pained, and so on. It is crucial for the image therapist to identify whatever the patient is feeling in order to be able to treat him. This method of diagnosis, which allows us to feel, see, and recognize the sensations of the patient, is called diagnosis by symptoms.

However, this alone is not enough since it is imperative for us to know the cause and the origins of the illness. For example, the symptom of reddening eyes can be explained in different ways. If you implement the use of diagnosis by symptoms, you would say that you experience discomfort around your eyes, pain, and, as anyone can see, a reddening of your eyes. Therefore, in regular medical practice, the doctor would search for what is wrong with your eyes.

In Traditional Chinese Medicine it is considered that red eyes are a sign of problems with the liver. In such an event, energy from the liver rises to the eyes and radiates through them. Once again, we see that TCM attempts to find the origin or roots of an illness that lie in a completely different organ than the eyes where we see the physical manifestation of the illness. Thus, in order to identify the origin of reddening eyes it is necessary to understand the cause-effect relationships.

And so, in IM we utilize several methods for diagnosis of illnesses:

- *The basic form of diagnosis—diagnosis with the hands.* With our hand we can conduct a physical and energetic diagnosis (you can sense warmth, heat, coldness, coolness, wind, numbness, etc); you can sense a pulse, whether it is fast or slow, strong or weak, on the surface or deep. Hands can detect even more precise information. Henceforth, in IM, if your hands are very sensitive, you can identify 80% of all illnesses. Physical sensations are stable and ever present. Whereas the Mind's eye or the Third eye may not always work, hands can always work and sense. Hands can also often be used to check that which we see with the Mind's eye.

- *Diagnosis by symptoms.* This method allows us to sense, see, and learn of the sensations felt by the patient. In IM, there is particular training that allows one to improve the sensitivity of a body healer. Upon contracting an illness, we experience physical and emotional sensations such as pain, heaviness, numbness, weakness, fever, nausea, and so on. Another form of sensations includes fear, depression, exhaustion, etc. Using your own body for diagnosis, you can sense and tell the patient what unpleasant sensation he is experiencing as well as in what organ or area he is experiencing them. Likewise, with the help of your body, you can understand the emotional condition of your patient.

- *Diagnosis through the questioning of the patient.* This method is not linked to receiving images. Except the regular questioning, used in western medicine and TCM, in IM, if you do not know the answer to a question you can ask it to the Teacher. This is referred to as *"the art of opening the spirit"*.

- *Diagnosis of the cause of the illness (Diagnosis with images).* This form of diagnosis presents itself as a method that allows one to identify the exact problem within the body in terms of seeing the disruption in the physical body, energy, and information of a patient. It can explain the physical condition of an individual and whether there are any stones, hernias, tumors, etc. that are affecting his physical structure or form. One can also see the condition and color of energy in various organs. The benefit of image therapy is that the viewing of images is an effective way of understanding the condition of the spirit and the cause of an illness which can be located outside the body. An image can show the connections between separate parts of the organism, the connections among inner organs, and connections with other people or any forms of life. A human is not alone; he is always connected to the Sky and the Earth. Many people's health is therefore impacted by events such as problems in the family, changes in the weather, and so on.

Another form of diagnosis implements the use of the Third Ear. Often, that which you can hear in reference to illness, you can also see with the help of the Third Eye. Within your body there is an array of biochemical reactions that occur. They are accompanied by light radiations and sounds. The ability to operate the Third Ear is received as a result of special training.

As a whole, the diagnostic methods of IM allows one to discover an image of the illness while the treatment methods of IM is the transformation of incorrect images to correct ones— the transformation of an ill individual to a healthy one.

Part Two

PRACTICAL APPLICATION

Chapter Three:
SELF HEALING

Self healing is a key aspect of IM. If we understand ourselves as well as the order and rules of life, then we can create conditions under which our body can heal itself. In general, our inner organism's capacity for self healing is very high.

To improve the sensitivity of our sensory organs and our diagnostic capabilities, one must cleanse the body and calm the mind. For this we can implement the use of a self healing method.

There are a large number of self healing methods but here we will discuss the simplest one. This method requires you to stand, relax, bring your mind to a state of serenity or quietness, and allow your body to move as it wills. You should not to be in control of your actions or to be thinking or analyzing anything—simply acknowledge your body's movements.

Often, your body begins to move in slow, fluid motions similar to those performed when stretching. We still do not fully understand the strength of our abilities and our self healing capabilities.

Self healing can be divided into two parts: part one—relaxing, part two—moving. Methods concerned with the ability to enter a state of silence and serenity are especially crucial for healing spiritual and energetic problems. Methods linked to movement are more commonly used for the treatment of physical illnesses.

For Example: You have acquired the flu. Stand up straight, relax, and your body will begin to move all by itself. You will soon begin to feel warmth and will sweat so much that the illness will depart your body along with the sweat.

This method can also be used to help treat patients. Following the diagnosis and discovery of the cause of the illness, you can, instead of treating the patient, present him with methods of self healing. You can explain and demonstrate exercises and meditations that are necessary for the treatment of his illness.

We can say that self healing is our first and last chance to improve our health. It is our first chance because it is the simplest thing to do. In certain cases it is our last chance as well because many illnesses still have no known cure, thus leaving methods of self healing as the only alternative. If you are being treated with the help of medical prescriptions or other alternative methods and are not seeing results, then you must use your own capabilities for regeneration.

In many cases, for the restoration of health you must first calm your mind and allow your body to begin the process on its own through the performance of actions that will be therapeutic for it. Self healing can be used to treat a patient of many illnesses.

Chapter Four:
METHODS OF HEALING
IN ENERGY MEDICINE

Image medicine tackles all kinds of problems in the body. We begin our studies from energy medicine that includes energy diagnosis and energy treatment or therapy. Ten special mantras, eight so called Big Methods, and four methods, or ways, of cleansing are used in this field.

BIG METHODS

The methods that have been deemed Big Methods are called thus because they can be used to treat not one type of illness but many types. They are equally effective in treating illnesses of the physical body as well as the energetic and informational systems.

Big Methods are simple but require constant practice in order to perfect and enhance them. If you begin by practicing a large amount of methods, then none of them will be effective. It is necessary to master either one or several methods because attempting to master all of them from the start is not possible.

In what cases and how do we implement the use of the Big Methods?

In certain cases a patient may experience a chronic pain, discomfort, and uncomfortable sensations, but these descriptions do not provide enough information to help determine the source of the problem on a physical level. In the process of diagnosis we would notice a dim color in his organs and other parts of the body as well insufficiently active energy flow at certain points. On the physical level, you note that the movement of the kidneys, intestines, and other organs is slowed. In this case, in order to restore the patient's health, it is necessary to use the *method of awakening*.

Method of Awakening

The first major method in IM is called the *Method of Awakening*. Let us analyze why it is given so much attention. The method of awakening fulfills three important functions:

- The awakening of the physical parts of organs or other body parts (such as the heart, liver, joint, etc.)
- The awakening of energy (in acupuncture this is called Sin Qi). This means that you must force improved work of your Qi.
- The awakening of shen and/or the mind.

This means that with the implementation of this method, we will awaken the physical body, the energy system, and the informational system. The theory of this method was described in ancient books and, in practice, I have found that certain organs, parts of the body, or functional systems do, in fact, sleep and thus must be awakened.

Why must we awaken our organs and individual cells?

Each cell in our body has a life of its own. Due to this, a cell may be in sleeping mode or in a bad emotional state. Inside our bodies, our organs, as a rule, have their own individual characteristics and personalities in the same way that people do. Sometimes we wish to sleep or sometimes we simply feel tired and do not want to do anything or sometimes we just do not wish to work and thus act lazy at our job. But what is the cause of these problems? How come our inner organs or cells may not want to work, fall asleep, or act lazy? This is similar to what occurs with our body as a whole: when we become tired, we require rest, and wish to sleep.

Prior to performing the awakening a diagnosis must be conducted in order to determine which cells are asleep. How do we determine whether cells are asleep? Well, how do we know that a person is asleep? With a person it easy to determine, through the use of one's regular sight, if a person, for example, is sleeping while the others are meditating. But to see sleeping cells within the body, one must use the Third Eye, or Eye of the Mind. Then we can discover that certain tissues, or muscles, or organs, or cells of the physical body are sleeping instead of working. As energy is concerned, under normal conditions, the energy is active and moves within us in a particular way. However, if the energy is sleeping then the movement is very weak and slow. If your Third eye is working then you can, at once, see the section in the body with the inactive energy. You can notice that a person's energy of fog or energy of light is weak and the work of the organ it is affecting is slower than usual.

If your Third Eye is not working, you can lead a diagnosis with your hands by checking various zones of the body with them. If a certain area is sleeping, then that area is more relaxed than those around it. If you are conducting a diagnosis through symptoms, then you connect yourself to the sensations of the patient and automatically feel the laziness, unwillingness to move, and exhaustion that he is experiencing. Regular medicine is unable to identify or explain these problems and, therefore, despite attempts to treat the seemingly unusual sensations, doctors continue being uncertain in the treatment methods they present. They may claim that such sensations are a result of kidney inflammation. However, blood analysis shows no abnormalities and the patient continues to feel very ill.

The reason behind this can be easily explained by the three components of our bodies: the problem can be energetic, physical, or spiritual. Of course, if a person is sick, he may sleep for an extended amount of time. A similar concept applies to our organs; they can sleep within our bodies longer than necessary for several reasons:

- As a result or side effect of a prescription medication
- As a result of disruption in one's emotional state

If, within your body, certain organs are asleep an abnormal amount of time, you may find that you experience the following symptoms: you may either wish to sleep more than necessary or you may have a disrupted sleep. Furthermore, in such cases, you become exhausted more easily; with a minimum amount of work completed you feel exhausted and are forced to take a break.

And so, *physical organs and cells* may, at times, be half asleep or lazy. This can be brought on by the consumption of large amounts of medication, pain killers, or sleeping pills. *Energy* can also sleep. Often, this phenomenon is associated with one's behavior in regular situations. For example, if a person has nothing to do, he may chose to sleep more than necessary and thus lead to decreased activity of his energy. Another factor that may impact your energy is your work. If your job requires you to remain in the same position with minimal movement for numerous hours then it may lead to a decrease in the activity of your energy as well. In certain cases, the *informational system* may sleep too. If in some area of the body your informational system has fallen asleep, then you will no longer be able to control that area of the body. The lack of control over a certain area of the body can lead to the appearance and growth of different and often dangerous cells. We can say that all cancer patients experience problems with the functionality of their informational systems. This means that, as a result of some external or internal factors, the informational system has fallen asleep and ceased working. If, for example, there is no control over the informational system of our heart because it has fallen asleep, then our hearts will begin working either too rapidly or too slowly. Furthermore, the sleep of a certain area of the informational system can affect the work of other organs or areas of the body and impair their functionality as well. *Shen (spirit and mind)* can fall asleep due to various reasons. As a rule, the sleeping of shen is linked to a person's emotions. There are situations in which you are forced to complete a task you do not wish to do and, as time passes, you become more and more unwilling to complete the task thus leading your spirit into a state of exhaustion and sleep. How do you know the state of your mind: awake, attempting to work, or already asleep? This is simple. If you are always tired while working, if you begin reading a book and promptly fall asleep, if you are always have difficulty concentrating or a bad memory, if you have slow reflexes—then your shen is definitely sleeping. Furthermore, if your shen is either asleep or lazy, you may even feel as though, despite being wide awake, your brain is not working as well or clearly as it should. Another example is as follows. A child is very active and does not differ in any way from his peers. However, when he goes to school, his activeness prevents him from learning because he is incapable of concentrating on anything specific. In this case as well we can say that the shen is asleep.

During my studies in school and college we had a lot of bad students and the predominant reason behind them being bad students is that their spirit was lazy and in a sleeping mode. Such cases are common—of students sitting in a class and seemingly listening yet at the same time it is as though they do not hear the teacher and are quick to fall asleep. Even when the teacher is addressing them and they open their eyes, it is as though they did not hear the question. This is explained by the fact that their spirit is asleep, their energy is asleep, and their physical body is asleep. If they remain in the same state for an extended amount of time, their brain can no longer actively work. In this case, the method of awakening can also be used. What does this entail?

The essence of the awakening method. If your child is sleeping but you need to awake her, what do you do? You quietly shake, stroke, and pat her while telling her "wake up". If we wish to wake up some organ, we use the same method. We activate our energy ball, through the "bigger-smaller" method, forcing it to pulsate and enter the sleeping or lazy area.

Awakening the physical organs

We will analyze this in reference to a liver. And so, if your liver is lazy or asleep, then you will place your hand with the energetic ball in that area, forcing it to pulsate within it, alternating between becoming larger and smaller (Picture 13). When the ball becomes larger, your hand is located on the surface of the body

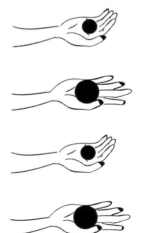

while the ball is inside, within the liver, and continues to pulsate. As the ball becomes larger, you mentally instruct your liver to "awake". The ball then becomes smaller and when it, once again, becomes larger, you instruct your liver to "awake" again before the ball decreases. With every time that the ball increases you tell your liver to awake, awake, awake, and even though your hand cannot reach inside the liver, your energy ball can.

If your child is fast asleep and despite your gentle attempts to wake her, continues to sleep and is nonresponsive, what do you begin to do? You begin to

Picture 13: Activating the Yin-Yang Ball

apply more strength to your actions. You stroke and shake her more intensely and continue to say "wake up, wake up". This method can also be applied to your work with the energy ball. With the ball in your hand, not only are you holding your hand over the ill area, forcing the ball to pulsate within it, and saying "awake, awake", but also are patting your hand over the area with the sick organ. As you pat your hand, the energy ball enters the organ and enlarges. As before, you mentally tell the organ to "awake, awake, awake..." every time the ball enters it.

Here, success is accomplished through the help of your mind and the vibrations of the energy ball in your hand. If you are incapable of awakening the organ, you will sense heaviness in that location. However, if you do manage to awake it, you will feel lightness and joy. If the organ is not awakening when you approach it nicely and lightly, then you must intensify your actions by patting harder and saying "awake" more seriously and forcefully. Intense awakening must occur in steps, not from the start, or else you risk damaging the organ. This is similar to waking a child, at first you try to do so quietly and calmly, and afterwards more and more intensely. If you begin waking the child as intensely as possible you may frighten her.

Experience shows that a similar method can be used to fix problems with the liver, with the kidneys, and so on. For example, the reason behind the chronic swelling of kidneys is often a decrease in their functionality. However, if we place our hand in the area of the kidneys and send energy pulsations alongside commands to "awake, awake", then the kidney immediately improve and, in a week, results are already visible.

Awakening Qi

In order to awaken Qi we apply the same exact method. We lay the patient down and begin patting him with our hand in the points of Yongquan, the exiting points of the kidneys' channels, on the bases of the feet. By patting the points in that way you are capable of awakening energy in the entire body. Afterwards, it is optimal to help the flow of energy from the feet upward by patting the legs of the patient from the bottom up. This method used to be considered very secretive since it is both very simple and accessible.

Awakening shen

The next big secret was the method by which shen, the mind and information, could be awakened. For the awakening of shen, several points around the area of the head are pressed by our fingers and vibrations. The first area is located a little above the point of Mingtang. If your shen is asleep then upon touching the area you will experience pain. With the help of your fingers you must press on that point for some time while repeating "awake, awake". There are two more points that are located behind the ears next to the point of Yuchen. Forthcoming books will describe other points that must be approached in a particular way in order to awaken one's shen.

It is important to note that when working with any patient it is vital that, at the first session, you must awake the physical body, then awake the energy, and at the end awaken his shen. Treatment of any illness can occur only after this is done. This way, after the first session, the patient will already feel better and stronger and, in turn, will trust you.

Still there is another form of treatment. I will describe *an example* of it. I had a patient who, during the duration of a year and a half, felt very ill, could not work, and slept a lot. Upon examination in a hospital, no problems were found because tests returned a normal chemical composition of her blood and a normal structure of her organ tissues. Still, it was obvious that she was sick. She had lost a lot of weight and her face had a stale and inactive color. During diagnosis I discovered that throughout her entire energy system Qi was moving listlessly but the cause of the problem was in her mind. Her liver as well was very weak and barely capable of moving. You can often determine the emotional condition of a person based on his liver— if a person is emotional than the energy in his liver moves very quickly whereas if he has little emotion then the liver's energy moves slowly. Through a conversation with her I found out that a year and a half ago she had a serious quarrel with her husband which resulted in him leaving her. She no longer saw him but has heard rumors that he had a new woman. This rumor only strengthened her depression. Previously, she and her husband had had a very good relationship and fought over insignificant things. However, their mutual inability to admit to their faults ultimately led to their separation.

I asked the husband's brother to write a letter to the woman in handwriting similar to that of her husband. The letter, delivered by a stranger in order to avoid sending it through the mail, described how her "husband" was writing to apologize, ask forgiveness for being wrong, and say he will shortly return. The wife believed the letter and shortly after receiving it she regained her energy, felt better, and, after a week, was completely back to normal.

This is an example of how to implement spiritual treatment. What is important in this case is that when an illness leaves, it usually does not return. For some time, the woman is happy and awaits her husband's return but, little by little, returns to her usual duties and normal state in the process.

However, in that situation the husband had left to work on a construction zone. His brother, inspired by the results of the treatment, found people to write a similar letter to the one that the wife had received and had it signed in the name of the wife. As a result, the husband returned home shortly before the Chinese New Year and brought the money with him. Both the woman and her husband were very happy since each thought the other apologized first. Eventually they found out the truth but forgave each other anyway and both came as guests to my Chinese New Year celebration.

In this example, the woman had no physical or energetic problem. Instead, as a result of her depressed emotional state, all her organs became very weak. In order to rid of such an illness it is essential to eradicate the cause.

And so, other than the method of awakening the area of energy medicine also provides us with other Big Methods to study.

Method of Regeneration

The second Big Method, the method of Regeneration (recovery), allows for the regeneration of cells of various tissues and organs such as muscle tissue, bone marrow, nerve fibers, liver cells, kidney cells, and so on. The principle of treating with this method is to change an incorrect image to a correct one.

Method of Substitution

The third Big method is the Method of Substitution. Our body is constructed in a way that many of its functions are duplicated. In the event that an organ in incapable of performing its specific function we develop the function in another organ capable of performing it, even if it is to a lesser extent. The purpose of the method of Substitution is to move the image of the organ that cannot perform a certain function well enough to another organ that can take onto itself the function through the implementation of substitution.

About these and other Big Methods you can read in subsequent books on IM.

MANTRAS

Mantra Hua 化

This mantra is used in order to destroy or melt bad substances located in our body that do not, in fact, belong to our bodies and must therefore be eradicated. For example, after any trauma, many dead blood cells remain in the area of the liver. Another example would be if you ate something that did not well with you. As a result, that substance remains in your liver, pancreas, or even kidneys for an extended amount of time. If any bad substance accumulates in these organs, you begin to feel heaviness or numbness in the area. Sometimes you may even experience a constant, long-lasting, dull, and blunt pain.

In such cases, Mantra Hua is implemented. The meaning of the mantra is to utilize the energy of a particular structure in order to "melt away" the illness. Your consciousness, thoughts, and energy thus change an ill area of the body into a healthy one.

The image you see must be as follows. You should see warmth, like that which is necessary for the melting of snow, radiating from your palm. Energy radiates from your palm and falls on and melts the bad substances within you in a similar fashion to a hot shower of water falling on and melting snow (Picture 14).

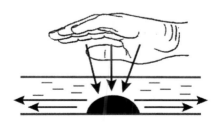

Picture 14: The Image of the Hua Mantra

What types of illness can be treated with Mantra Hua?

1. This mantra can be used to treat problems with blood. Whether a person has high cholesterol, cholesterol plaques, viscous blood, or problematic circulation through narrow veins, the mantra can lead to the restoration of proper blood functionality. If there are problems with circulation, you must direct the mantra at your liver. For this, you must first place your hand in the area of your liver and sense that you have touched the liver or came in contact it. Meanwhile, you must sense the energy moving from your hands and intermingling with the energy of your liver. As a result, you should feel heaviness depart from the liver and a feeling of lightness appear.

2. This mantra can also be used before and after a heart attack or stroke. A good doctor is able to notice and prevent the illness. On the other hand, a bad doctor will not be able to uncover it. This mantra is capable of preventing both because it causes the melting of cholesterol plaques in blood and the widening of veins that have narrowed in places.

3. Lastly, this mantra is also useful when it comes to flu-like illnesses. If you have become infected with the flu or a virus, then bad substances inevitably collect in your lungs and cause you to develop a cough. Often, you are left coughing them up for a long time after contracting the illness. Here, too, you can use Mantra Hua, this time around the lung and bronchial tube area, in order to accelerate the eradication of the mucus and ultimate recovery from the illness.

The reading of a mantra should be smooth rather than abrupt. In order for a mantra to have its proper effect it is also necessary to practice it. Practice not only improves the effectiveness of the mantra but also your understanding of its purpose and meaning. Without working with the mantra and attempting to operate it, you cannot hope to understand it. In most cases, the reading of a mantra requires no more than five minutes; though sometimes as much as a half hour is needed. This mantra is useful only for the soft materials within the body—the body's solid materials require other mantras.

Other Mantras

As we mentioned previously, in total, ten mantras are used in IM. Among them, other than Mantra Hua, are those mentioned below.

1. **Mantra Tong ("Open").** This mantra is used if a confined area of an energy channel is blocked. Using this mantra we move the energy of a point prior to the block to a point after the blocked area. In this way the channel is cleaned and unblocked. For the mantra to work properly, it must be pronounced in a way that causes vibrations in the organ. This means that you must detect and select a proper frequency for the mantra to obtain a desired result. To correctly use sounds and actions linked to vibration and shaking, we must be well aware of the physiology and rhythm with which the organ operates. You must understand how to impact the organ in a more forceful fashion. The sounds of the mantra must travel with the energy deeply into the area with which you are working.

2. **Mantra Xiao ("Destroy").** This mantra is designated to work with different solids that occur in the body, such as swelling, stones, and tumors. This mantra is not ef-

fective enough on cancerous tumors though, so a different-ent mantra is used in those cases. The main uses of this mantra are to break up stones and treat benign tumors.

明 3. **Mantra Ming ("Bright").** This mantra is used for the awakening of energy and shen as well as for the cleansing and brightening of the body and its energy.

大 4. **Mantra Zhang.** This mantra is used for the improvement of circulation of blood and energy in the body as well as the widening of necessary areas, parts of the body, channels, and so on.

小 5. **Mantra Shuo.** The effects of this mantra are opposite those of the previously mentioned Mantra Zhang. It is used to remove swelling which results from increasing the size of areas of the body. This mantra can only be used on areas free from any infections.

走 6. **Mantra Zou ("Go").** This mantra is implemented to help with some of the body's movements.

变 7. **Mantra Bian ("Change").** This mantra is used when it is necessary to change an image within someone.

You can acquire more information about these and other mantras in subsequent books or at seminars with the Master.

BEIJING'S MEDICAL-RESEARCH INSTITUTE "KUNDAWELL"

Created, founded, and directed
by Professor of TCM Mingtang Xu

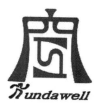

Today, the Beijing institute "Kundawell" performs several different actions.

Research programs include the study of difficult and untreatable illnesses, a search for the causes of these illnesses, as well as a complex treatment of these illnesses through the methods of Qigong Therapy, IM, and TCM. The main advantage of this treatment is that it approaches the patient from three different aspects: physical body, energy, and information. IM's mission is not to find and treat the symptoms but rather the underlining cause of a patient's illness.

Wellness programs include the diagnosis and development of self healing techniques through the methods of Qigong Therapy, IM, TCM, and meditation.

Educational programs work at preparing qualified image therapists and family health nurses capable of operating the methods of IM and following a specified medical diet. The program of study includes the mastery of the fundamental theories, methods of diagnosis and treatment according to IM, study of the basic information and methods of traditional Chinese and western medicine, and practical lessons with skilled specialists. These studies are intended for two months, a year, two years, three years, or four years.

The institute also works at developing *herbal remedies*, and *the study and combining of effective and natural methods for health restoration*.

Website:
www.kundawell.com or http:/www.kundawell.cn/english

Contacts:
Personal research programs: research@kundawell.com
Study: education@kundawell.com
Wellness programs: wellness@kundawell.com
For cooperation and general questions: infor@kundawell.com

Made in the USA
Lexington, KY
22 August 2012